KNOW ALL ABOUT THE HUMAN METABOLISM

-

A FACTUAL GUIDE ABOUT YOUR BODY SYSTEM LIKE YOU'VE NEVER SEEN BEFORE

INTRODUCTION

The human body is a simple yet complex structure. Thanks to modern science and technology, we have learned so much about how our body works. Every time you slurp a smoothie or swallow some soup, your body works tirelessly to process all the nutrients you have eaten. After your food is digested, all the nutrients you have eaten become the fuel and building blocks needed by your body. The body gets the energy required from food through this process called metabolism.

Metabolism is pronounced as *muh-TA-buh-lih-zum.* It is a collection of all chemical reactions that occur in the body's cells. This process converts fuel in the meals we eat into energy which is needed to power our activities, from moving to reasoning to growing. Some specific proteins in our bodies control the reactions of metabolism. Each chemical reaction is organized with other functions of the body. In fact, lots of metabolic reactions occur at the same time to maintain the health of our cells.

Metabolism is a continual process, and it begins when we start developing in out mother's wombs and ends when our hearts stop. It is a significant process for every life form — not just humans. If the metabolism process stops, living things die. Consider this example of how metabolism works in humans as well as how it begins with plants. In the first place, a green plant absorbs energy from sunlight. This plant uses the energy and a molecule which is called chlorophyll (it gives plants their bright green color) to use water and carbon dioxide to build sugars. This process is known as photosynthesis. You may have learned about this term in biology class.

When animals and people eat the plants (if they're carnivores, and they eat animals that have consumed the plants), they consume this energy (in the form of sugar), with other vital chemicals for cell-building. The body's next phase is to break down the sugar so that the released energy can be distributed and used as fuel to power the body's cells.

After you eat the food, molecules in the body's digestive system which are called enzymes break these proteins down into what is called amino acids. The fats are also broken down into fatty acids, while the carbohydrates are converted into simple sugars such as glucose. As well as sugar, both fatty acids and amino acids can be used by the body as energy sources when needed.

Such compounds are then absorbed into the blood and are transported to the cells. When they enter the cells, enzymes act to accelerate or regulate the chemical reactions that are involved with "metabolizing" these compounds. The energy gotten from these compounds are released for use or stored in the body tissues, especially the muscles, liver, and body fat.

The entire process of metabolism is a balancing act that involves two kinds of activities occurring at the same time. Some of the activities involve;

- Anabolism is pronounced as *uh-NA-buh-lih-zum.* It is also constructive metabolism, and is all about storing and building. It supports growth of new cells, storage of energy for future use and maintenance of the body tissues. During anabolism, the small molecules are converted into larger, and more complex molecules of fat, carbohydrate, and protein.
- Catabolism is pronounced as *kuh-TA-buh-lih-zum.* It is also called destructive metabolism, and it is a process that produces the energy which is needed for all cell activity. During this process, the cells break down large the molecules to release energy. The energy release provides some fuel for anabolism and heats the body. It allows the muscles to contract so the body can move.

When complex chemical units are converted into more simple substances, a waste product released during catabolism are removed from the kidney, skin, lungs, and intestines.

Different hormones of the body's endocrine system play a part in regulating the rate of metabolism. Thyroxine which is pronounced as thigh-ROK-seen is a hormone which is produced and is also released from the thyroid gland. It helps determines how slow or fast the chemical reaction of metabolism happens in a person's body. Another gland which is called the pancreas secretes hormones that also help determine whether the body's primary metabolic activity during a particular period will be catabolic or anabolic. For instance, after eating, usually more anabolic activity happens because eating increases the body's level of glucose in the blood. Well, this is just the beginning of a fascinating journey into the metabolism world. In this book, you will learn all you need to know about how your body metabolism works in an interesting and straightforward way. Happy Reading!!!

CHAPTER ONE
THE HUMAN METABOLISM

We always talk about metabolism like it is something we can control by running faster, downing some green tea, or gulping a pill. You've seen the articles headlined "Boost your metabolism" or "Try this high-metabolism diet to slim down." But this hides many truths concerning this vital, yet somewhat mysterious, biological process. Here are some facts about your metabolism;

- **Your metabolism is in all cells in your body**

Like it's a muscle or organ somehow or that they can flex control lots of folks talk about their metabolism. But in reality, your metabolism refers to a series of chemical processes in each cell that turn the calories you eat into fuel to keep you alive. The primary organs of the body — liver, the brain, kidneys, and heart — account for about half of the energy burned at rest, while fat, the digestive system, and notably the body's muscles account for the remainder.

- **Size Determines our Metabolic Need**

The thought that smaller and thinner individuals have a quicker basal metabolic rate or the ability to burn off calories is false. In fact, the body size and composition determines how much fuel (or food nutrients) you will require in order to produce enough energy to function. In essence, the bigger you are; the more food nutrients you will need to function.

- **Most of the energy you burn off is from your resting metabolism**

There are three primary ways your body burns energy each day: 1) the resting, or basal, metabolism — energy used for your body's basic functioning; 2) the energy used to break down food (also called the thermic effect of food); and The energy used in physical action.

- **Metabolism can vary a lot between individuals, and scientists are not sure why.**

It's true that two individuals with the same size and body composition can have completely different metabolisms. One of them can have huge meal after huge meal and gain no weight, while the other has to count calories to prevent weight gain. Researchers have found some factors that determine how fast a man's metabolism will be. Included in these are the amount of lean muscle and fat tissue in the body, age, and genetics (though researchers do not know why some families have higher or lower metabolic rates).

Since women with any given body makeup and age burn fewer calories than comparable men, sex also matters in this context. You cannot easily measure your metabolic rate in an accurate way (there are some commercially available tests, but the best measurements come from research studies that use high-priced equipment like a metabolic chamber). However, you can get a rough estimate of your metabolic rate by putting some basic data into on-line calculators. It'll inform you how many calories you are expected to burn off daily, and if you eat that many and your weight stay the same, it's likely correct.

- **Another thing that slows down the metabolism: becoming old**

The effect happens gradually, even if you've got the same amount of muscle and fat tissue. So when you are 60, you burn fewer calories than when you're 20.

This drop begins as young as age 18 — and why this occurs is also another metabolism question researchers have not answered.

- **You cannot really speed up your metabolism for weight loss**

There is a lot of hype around "speeding up your metabolism" and losing weight by exercising more to build muscle, eating different foods, or taking supplements. But it is really very hard to do. While there are particular foods — like fruits, chili, and other spices — that may speed the basal metabolic rate up, the change is so minimal and short lived; it'd never have an impact on your own waistline.

Building more muscles may be slightly more helpful. Here's why; one of the factors that change your metabolic rate is the quantity of lean muscle you've got. At any given weight, the more muscle in your body, and the fat, the higher your metabolic rate. That is because muscle uses a lot more energy than fat while at rest. So the logic is if you reduce your body fat, and can build up your muscle, you'll have a higher metabolism and fast burn the fuel within your body. But there's a caveat if you've got more muscle, it burns fuel more quickly. But that's only half the question. If you do gain more muscle and efficiently speed up your metabolism, you have to fight the natural inclination to eat more as an effect of your higher metabolism.

Many people give in to the hunger that ends up adding more fat along with the muscle.

- **Dieting can slow down your metabolism**

While it is extremely hard to speed the metabolic rate up, researchers have found there are things people do can slow it down — like severe weight reduction programs. For years, various researchers have been studying a phenomenon which is called "metabolic adaptation" or "adaptive thermogenesis." This theory suggests that as individuals lose weight, their basal metabolic rate — the energy used for the basic functioning when the body is at rest — really slows down to a greater degree than would be anticipated from the weight loss.

To be clear: The body is subsequently smaller, and it makes sense that losing weight will slow down the metabolism a bit, since by slimming down, muscle loss is involved and does not have to work as hard every minute to keep running.

CHAPTER TWO
HOW DOES METABOLISM WORK?

Metabolism is a chemical process that is complicated, so it's weird that many folks think of it in its simplest sense: as something that affects how easily our bodies gains weight or slims down. A calorie can be referred to as a unit that measures how much energy a special food supplies to the body. One chocolate bar has more calories than a single apple, so it supplies more energy — to the body. Just as a car keep gas in the gas tank until it is needed to fuel the engine, the body stores calories — mainly as fat. When you overfill your car's gas tank, it will spill over onto the sidewalk. Likewise, if someone eats too many calories, they "spill over" excess fat in the body.

The amount of calories a person burns in a day is impacted by how much that individual exercises, the quantity of fat and muscle in her or his body, as well as their basal metabolic rate. This basal metabolic rate, or BMR, is a measure of the speed at which someone's body "burns" energy while at rest. This BMR can play a role in a person's predisposition to weight gain. For instance, a person with a low BMR (who consequently burns fewer calories while at rest or sleeping) will tend to gain more pounds of body fat over time, compared with a similar-sized person with an average BMR who eats the same quantity of food and gets the same quantity of exercise.

What factors determine an individual's BMR? To a certain extent, people's basal metabolic rate is inherited — passed on through the genes of his or her parents. Occasionally health problems can change someone's BMR. But individuals can alter their BMR in some ways. For instance, exercising more will not only cause someone to burn more calories directly from the additional task itself but by becoming more physically healthy, BMR will be increased. BMR is, in addition, affected by body composition — people with more muscle and less fat generally have higher BMRs.

Things That Can Go Wrong with Metabolism

Most of the time your metabolism functions effectively without any. But sometimes a person's metabolism can cause major issues such as a metabolic disorder. In a general sense, a metabolic disorder is any disease that's caused by an abnormal chemical reaction in the cells of the body. When the metabolism of the body chemicals is faulty or blocked, it can cause a buildup of hazardous substances in the body or a deficiency of materials needed for normal body function, either of which can lead to serious health issues.

THE METABOLISM OF AN ATHLETE

It is widely known that sports make for better overall fitness of the body and increased metabolic rates. Routine exercises, done or at least 3 or 4 times each week, can help people's bodies become more efficient in the way they burn fats.

Professional athletes have far better metabolic rates than regular folks, just because years and years of training have altered their bodies in a way which allows it to quickly digest and convert a lot of nutrients, for the maximum output of energy, at any given time. A long-distance runner, for example, has the entire body perfectly adapted for this kind of course. He uses just about the same number of energy at all time, and his muscular fibers are used, over long amounts of time, for a sustained effort. On the other hand, short-distance runners, who rely on rate, have a body that is used to having everything drained out of it in a very brief outburst, as in a 100 meter (330 feet) sprint.

Yale University scientists who were led by Professor Douglas Befroy stated that muscle mitochondria is responsible for the performance of sportsmen, which are cell components very much like energy converters – these burn fats and sugars in the cell and generate energy-carrying ATP molecules. These will provide the muscles with increased oxygen-processing capabilities. Finally, the effect of mitochondria is the skill the muscles have, of working better for more.

The researchers also discovered that professional sportsmen also burn more energy when they are resting or sleeping, not only during active periods. This implies that the excess energy is lost and the one created by mitochondria is transformed into heat. Discoveries like this one are essential for the field of medicine because they could direct the way to better understanding how severe diseases, like diabetes, work and perhaps even discover some potential treatments.

What athletes say about the metabolism?

Nancy Lieberman who was a professional basketball player stated that nutrition plays a role in the function of the metabolism. Despite the fact that some people are blessed with a faster metabolism, an unhealthy diet can worsen it. She said she tries to eat only balanced diet which contains vegetables, healthy meats, and fruits. She has never been on a specific diet and doesn't even count her calories, she just listens to her body and gives it what it needs.

Another athlete, a marathoner named Mike Wardian spoke about the workings of his system. He said that he only picked a diet that worked for him and not just a specialized diet. He ate lots of carbs, fruits, bread, pasta, dairy and nut butter, but excluded meat from the diet. This his personalized diet gave him energy while accelerating his metabolism.

Ben Greenfield who was a triathlete also found a way to manipulate his metabolism. He stated that he followed a strict high fat, carbohydrate diet and restricts himself 5 days in a week to less than 100g or 200g at most of the carbs. When you force our body to rely only on fatty acids to fuel the body, you offer steady fuel for your brain, and this prevents you from being weak during a prolonged exercise session. You also increase your insulin sensitivity as well as your blood sugar stabilization. This lets you avert energy crashes and nerve damage or blood vessel damage from high sugar levels. You also spare protein from being utilized as energy, which preserves a lean muscle mass. Lastly, you decrease lactic acid production while increasing pH, both of which lessen net acidity in our bodies.

Joel Runyon, a Super Triathlete also said that he tries to eat as much "healthy food" as possible. To be precise, he tried to cut out processed junk as much as possible. Usually, it falls within a paleo diet framework. Because of the variety of things, he does, he tends to eat different things, but this depends on the specific task at hand. For instance, his diet when he's working on sustaining six pack abs is significantly different from when he's training for any ultra-marathon. He believes that in the end it all really depends on the goals people set, but he finds that eating as much healthy food as possible helps."

CHAPTER THREE

HOW THE METABOLISM AFFECTS THE BODY

Your body needs the energy to operate. However, you can alter the way your body uses energy. If you do it right, you can control your weight. Metabolism is the complex procedure by which nutrients are broken down by our body and creates and uses energy. It's also what makes it possible for our hearts our brains to work, and our lungs to be filled with air. In a nutshell, metabolism is what keeps our bodies working.

- **The energy you need**

Every one metabolizes in different ways. Some folks' speed is slower, and some of us have a faster metabolic rate. Some people burn up the calories they use up more rapidly than others. Each of us has distinct energy needs too. Most are used for basic functions—like pumping blood—that occur regardless of what you're doing. The quantity of energy used for these fundamental functions is known as your basal metabolic rate (BMR). (To estimate your BMR, multiply your weight in pounds by 10.)

Typically, your BMR represents about 60 percent of your overall daily calorie needs, based on the school. Of 30 percent are needed for powering, 10 percent for digestion and the physical action itself. You'll gain weight if you consume more calories than your body uses up. However, you can take steps to "rev up" your metabolism and burn off extra calories before they're stored as fat. Understanding the variables that determine your metabolic rate—both favorably and negatively—is a great starting point.

Variables that are unchangeable

Specific variables influencing metabolism are beyond your control. Among these are;

- **Age**: Teens and children need more calories per pound than adults because they're growing and need fuel. Usually, as we age, our action level declines. All this leads to a fall in energy and BMR needs.

- **Genetics:** Just as family ties can affect your well-being and risk for illness, your metabolism can be influenced by them.

- **Sex and Body size**: The heavier you're, the more energy it requires. Needless to say, you can adjust your weight. But this is one reason why guys, who have more muscle and frequently weigh more than women, usually need more calories.

- **Height:** Height isn't changeable, and it comes into play also. The body of a tall man loses more heat because of this and has more surface area than a short man. Thus, modulating body temperature—another procedure fueled by basal metabolism—needs more energy.

- **Hormone imbalance.** The American College of Sports Medicine reports that thyroid hormones, which basically tells your body's cells how many calories to burn off, usually become less effective in people after age 40.

A WORD FOR DIETERS

There are specific foods that can boost metabolism. And you might learn of them being connected with specific diets or diet products. Cayenne pepper and green tea are two examples. The following chapters would expand more on metabolism building foods. The effects of these items aren't long lasting. Anyone who's trying to get a metabolism push from supplements or pills must be mindful as these products may cause side effects. Do you really need to drop pounds? The best tip is to work out and eat healthily. They'll boost your metabolism and also result in successful weight loss.

CHAPTER FOUR
SLOW METABOLISM VS. FAST METABOLISM: WHICH IS PECULIAR TO YOU?

Remember that metabolism refers to the body's chemical process which is responsible for sustaining basic body functions like breathing, digestion, and building cells. These reactions require energy that is gotten from calories in food. Your body metabolic rate is the number of calories required to maintain these essential functions. The main difference between a slow and fast metabolism lies in how many calories the body needs to function. Fast metabolism always burns more calories than a slow one. Things that determine the metabolic rate include; body composition, gender, daily activities, age, and genetics.

Basal metabolic rate(the rate at which your body uses energy when you are resting to maintain all vital functions like; breathing and keeping warm), daily activity and thermic effect (the amount of energy used that is above the resting metabolic rate. It is usually due to what is spent on processing food for storage and use) are the three major factors that affect an individual's metabolic rate.

The basal metabolic rate burns about 40-70% of a person's daily calorie intake. When a person has a slow metabolism, it is usually because the basal metabolic rate is slow. Every one hundred calories an individual consumes typically requires at least ten calories to digest- this is the thermic effect of the food you eat. Your physical activities on the other hand also burn off calories, - the energy required to get out of bed, and power work out.

SLOW METABOLISM

If you are adding weight while you are eating the same food you've been eating for decades, then it's possible that your metabolism is slowing down. Your muscle burns more calories than your fat tissue. As you grow older, you will be less active, and your calorie-burning muscle would turn into fat. This would subsequently slow down your metabolic rate. This is also one of the reasons why females generally have slower metabolisms than men; women genetically have less muscle. Not eating enough calories can also make your metabolic rate slow down. According to a research published by the

University of Illinois, eating less slows down your metabolism by 30%.

How to know when your metabolism is slow

- Losing weight is far more difficult than gaining it

The feeling you get when your old weight loss tricks lead to dead ends can be frustrating. Trying to lose weight with methods that have worked for you in the past, but getting little or no results. This is one of the indicators that your metabolic rate has slowed down.

- You can't bring yourself to lose weight no matter what type of exercise you do

For many years, people have believed that losing weight simply revolves around calories. So it doesn't really matter what you eat as long as the calories get burnt off. Well, if you must know, some people run more than ten miles a day and still don't lose weight. So practically, it not just about the calories. It's more about the foods you put into your system.

When you notice that you can't lose weight no matter how much you work out, then your metabolism is slow. Exercises in collaboration with a healthy diet can help boost your metabolic rate.

- You can gain weight even when you eat very little

When you place yourself on a severely strict diet, your body goes into a mode known as "survival mode". Because your body is not getting enough food to go on, it starts storing anything it sees just in case. This is actually a defense mechanism. So your body is trying to save your life.

Rather than using food for fuel, your body stores fat for future use. So if you want your efforts to pay off, you have to feed your body and your metabolism to lose weight. All you have to do is feed your body with the right food. Eat things that stoke your metabolic fire.

- You start noticing fat in areas you've never had it before

Almost everyone has trouble spots- those bulges where you always gain and lose weight. However, when you start noticing fat in new areas, your metabolism is probably slowing down. Your body is desperately searching for new areas to store up fat.

When you start seeing fat in your midsection, it could mean that your cortisol (the hormone that gives your body the order to store fat in your tummy) are out of control. This usually happens when you are stressed, and your metabolism is over tasked.

- You start getting cellulite in new places

40% of women (physically fit women included) have cellulite on the upper thigh, backs, buttocks, and hips. However, when you start to noticing cellulite in places you ordinarily didn't, your metabolism could be slowing down. The cellulitis appears when your body starts searching your muscles desperately for fuel; soft fatty deposits are left behind. These are cellulitis. You also start losing collagen and elastin. This usually leaves your skin looking stretchy. It can also make cellulite more noticeable, and your body starts looking fatter.

- When your heels are cracked and dry and, you are losing hair

Your thyroid is not just responsible for your metabolic health; it is also responsible for healthy hair and healthy skin. Some indicators of slow metabolism include; hair loss, cracked skin or even dry skin. In women, these things may also indicate a hormonal imbalance.

- You have uncontrollable afternoon sugar cravings

It is your adrenal gland that is responsible for telling your body to release fat for fuel, especially in the afternoon. When this happens, your blood sugar drops and your body starts giving signs. It pushes you to eat something sugary. The problem arises because sugary food doesn't provide you with the required energy for a long do they wouldn't keep you going for long. When your metabolism is fast, it can properly regulate your blood sugar and give you energy through the day.

Things that you subconsciously or consciously do to ruin your metabolism

- Midnight snacking is the number one killer of your metabolism. Even when you feel hungry, drink a glass of water and go back to sleep. To avoid waking up to eat in the middle of the night, try and eat dinner four hours before you sleep.
- You don't sleep well enough at night. When you deprive yourself of sleep, you slow down your metabolism unknowingly.
- You don't drink enough water, especially in the morning. You're simply dehydrating yourself and slowing your metabolism. Drink a glass of water every morning.
- Drinking too much caffeine can slow down your metabolic rate.
- You don't take enough fruits.
- You don't eat organic meals.
- You totally avoid carbs.
- You lost weight too fast.

- You do not eat any nuts because you're scared nuts are fatty.
- You hardly engage in any physical activity.
- You do not eat organic meals.
- You don't work out at the right time.
- You consume way too many pesticides.
- You consume dairy toxins in processed foods.
- When you drink water with too much chlorine and fluoride.
- You always take unnecessary medications.
- You do not get enough protein. We already talked about the importance of protein in boosting a metabolism.
- You don't consume enough calories.
- You eat tiny servings.
- You don't take in enough vitamin D.
- You don't take in enough calcium.
- You eat too much of refined carbs.
- You do not take probiotics.
- You eat too many sweets.
- You take way too much alcohol.
- You sit around all day long doing nothing.
- You consume too many calories late in the day.
- You take sea salt instead of table salt.
- You work at night all the time.

- You eat odd meals at odd times.

FAST METABOLISM

If you are an individual blessed with a fast metabolism, then you would be privileged to eat anything you want and still look fighting fit. Genetics play a major role this case. Muscular men are more likely to have a hereditary higher metabolism. Although high calorie burning could be due to work out. Building muscle and working out pays off as it speeds up your metabolic rate. This is why bodybuilders and athletes usually eat more food but hardly ever get fat.

The fact remains that you can always learn to speed up your metabolism. There are lots of foods that can help you boost your metabolism including;

- Blueberries.
- Almonds
- Whey Protein.
- Salmon.
- Psyllium Husk.
- Spinach
- Turkey.
- Oatmeal.
- Green tea.
- Water.

Every human has a unique metabolic type, so it is important that we all learn how to eat the right food according to our metabolic type. The same foods that make you fat may keep your friends slim. You gave to be very careful if you want to achieve your goals. You can check your metabolic type online from authority website that allows people test their metabolic type.

You can also run a blood test to find out your unique metabolic rate. This would require you see your doctor who would give you his recommendation afterward. It is important that you find out if your metabolism is fast or slow before you start trying to work on it.

CHAPTER FIVE

HOW TO KICK START SLOW METABOLISM

When you are cutting calories especially to lose weight, it's important that you don't go too low. Consuming anything less than 1200 calories for ladies and 1800 for men may slow down the metabolic rate. Increase your calories a little to increase your metabolism. Adding muscles to your frame will give your metabolism a boost. Try strength-training at least two times a week. You can use free weights or do body resistance exercises like squats, push-ups, and lunches. This would all help boost your metabolism by building your calorie-burning muscles. Engaging in cardiovascular exercises (high-intensity workouts that increase the heart rate) are an excellent way to kick-start your metabolism.

You should find more days to be active. Increase your daily walk to 39-60 minutes. Walking around your office from time to time can help too. Pace when you're making a call. Stand at the counter when you want to type letters and emails.

Metabolism boosters

- **Building muscle:** Muscle burns more energy than fat. So altering fat into muscle can help you burn off more calories at rest. Research has found that for every pound of muscle we take, we're burning off about six calories, whereas, for every pound of fat we take, about two calories burn off.

- **Being energetic all day:** Metabolism is accelerated better if you're energetic through the day in 10-minute exercises rather than just spending one hour at the fitness center.

- **Eating more frequently**: Try eating more generally—but not more food. Snacks each day and several small meals are better than three big meals.

If you can consume the right types of foods every few hours, you will have a constant amount of energy, and your body will rev up and burn off those calories too.

- **Eating the right things:** Giving some thought to what you'll eat is significant also. Carbs are most people's primary energy source, but the body works to process protein. Your metabolic rate may actually improve if you have protein with carbs. Good carbs include yogurt; vegetables; fruits; and whole grain bread, pasta, cereal, and crackers. Examples of wholesome proteins contain eggs, fish, thin chicken, legumes, tofu and peanut butter.

- **Not skipping meals:** you're essentially sending a signal to your brain that you're in starvation mode when you skip meals. Metabolism slows to help you to survive because the body isn't sure when it is going to get food again.

Some specific ways to kick start your metabolic rate include;

- Eating with your non-dominant hand or using chopsticks
If you are regularly right handed, eating with your left hand or with chopsticks will help slow down your eating speed. This will help you chew smaller bites. These two things would work together to reduce your food intake and ultimately help reduce body weight. Serving meals on smaller plates and bowls will help you consume less.

- Place your food far from the table
Serving food directly from the counter will help reduce your desire to eat a second plate. The fact that your food is not in front of you would reduce your appetite for more. You'll also be acutely aware of how much you've eaten.

- Slow down and chew more

Slow down and chew your food, even more, would give your brain time to sync with your stomach. It should take approximately twenty to thirty minutes for your stomach to send the necessary signals to your brain. The signal is meant to tell the brain that you are full. When you eat too fast, you don't give your body enough time to register the food, and you're subsequently overeating.

- Eat before you leave your home

Whenever you have an event to attend, it's important that you eat before you leave the house. When you know that refreshments would be served at the event, you shouldn't look forward to eating there. Eating before you love would thus help curb the desire to eat even when the food is free and appetizing.

- Eat snacks in between meals

If you are going to take snacks with you, you should put them in one serving packs, not large bags. The bigger the container, the more you eat. The smaller the container, the lower your consumption. Try as much as possible to avoid jumbo size containers as they only encourage you to eat more.

- Eat before you eat your normal meal

Before you eat your regular meal, eat a small portion of a healthy snack or a salad. This would help you feel more satisfied, and it would eliminate cravings.

- When eating out, avoid bread and request for a take-home container

Before you start eating, pack up a little portion of your meal and bring it home for another meal. Restaurant portions are more likely to be bigger than homemade meal portion. Bringing a small portion home would help reduce how much you eat.

- Occupy your mouth and hands when watching a movie

Chewing gum and squeezing stress balls are two good ways to occupy your mouth and hand. Rather than reaching for chips or any other junk, this would be a good way to keep busy while watching the TV. If possible, avoid food commercials. They subconsciously trigger you to reach for food.

- Substitute junk food for healthy meals

Try and alternate junk for healthier foods. For instance, you can eat frozen grapes if you're having Popsicle cravings. You can also substitute a bowl of ice cream for yogurt and blueberries.

Speed Up Your Metabolism Using Meal Time Management

- Don't skip breakfast

When we sleep, our metabolism slows down a great deal. It would only go back to normal after you've had your first meal. So skipping breakfast isn't a good idea if you're trying to boost your metabolic rate. It's true that your body will burn a few calories when you skip breakfast. However, you'll still have enough energy to go through the day or until your next meal. On the other hand, when you eat up to 350 calories in the morning, you jumpstart your metabolism instantly and keep it burning all day long.

You can eat high fiber carbs like grain cereals, fruits, and egg whites. When compared to fats, these foods take more time to be absorbed by the body. This means you'll not get hungry fast and you'll avoid overeating during your next meal.

Try to avoid midnight snacks, in particular before bedtime. This is because you don't engage in any physical activity in your sleep. Remember that food is meant to serve as energy and when it doesn't serve as energy, it converts to fat. Eat light meals for dinner and save up your bulk appetite for the next day.

- Eat all day. Yes all day long

You may not have known this but eating 5 to 6 small meals a day is much better than eating three large servings. Don't worry; you'll not gain weight. Eating smaller portions several times would help improve digestion and boost overall metabolic rate. Eating past six doesn't make you gain weight. You can decide to savor a healthy meal about four hours before you sleep.

Eat one small meal every three to four hours a day. Add more proteins especially for dinner and lunch. Things like chicken, fish, legumes and tuna are perfect sources of protein. Your metabolic rate would increase, and your body would burn off more calories. Protein is harder to break down than carbohydrates so your body would burn off more calories.

Add a little pepper to your dinner soup or tofu. Spices actually heighten your resting metabolic rate temporarily by secreting more stress hormones. More of jalapeno and cayenne peppers help burn more calories.

Eating extra spicy meals tends to make you feel full faster even if you have only consumed half your plate. Do not forget to maintain your low-fat meal before you order a box of Indian curry or even Bicol Express.

Speed up Your Metabolic Rate by Counting Calories

It is true that nobody really likes crunch numbers, particularly during meals. Notwithstanding, calorie counting is an amazing way to keep track of your fitness level and improve your metabolic rate. Keep in mind that your body will typically try to normalize your system, even your weight. When you start removing 1,000 calories from your diet, your body would respond by slowing down your metabolic rate because it assumes that you are starving. This is the defense mechanism that was mentioned in the previous chapter.

There is no clear cut rule when it comes to determining the number of calories your body needs to take in daily. This is not an exact science. So you should reduce your calorie intake, but only in moderation and don't ever do anything radical to your diet.

Speed up Your Metabolism With Water Therapy

It sounds simple, but in reality, many people take drinking lots water for granted. Your metabolism needs lots of water to digest food. If you want to boost your metabolic rate, you have to drink more water. Drink no less than eight glasses of water a day. If you do heavy exercises, then add an extra cup or two. Don't make a habit of drinking cocktail or beer during meals.

Take water, not alcohol. Drinking lots of water makes up about 60% of your body. Alcohol also causes you eat more. Whenever you drink alcohol, your body burns the alcohol first. The meal becomes nothing but fat.

At least now you know how beer belly is formed.

Use exercise to boost your metabolic rate

A physical fitness program is never complete without the right volume of exercise. Nobody likes to do it, but everybody needs; fat and slim alike. Weightlifting significantly increases your metabolism, even when you are doing nothing. When you possess enough muscle density, you can burn no more than 100 calories simply by watching television alone.

Diet always goes with the right amount of exercise. Both are essential if you are to achieve your health and fitness goals. You muscle burns off more calories than fat. The truth is that running endlessly in one place may not get you far either. Try and combine cardiovascular activities, diet, and intense strength workouts if you want to boost your metabolism. The weight you lose should be from fat, and not from muscles.

Boost your metabolism by relaxing

Finally, something that seems easy! Getting sufficient sleep say; seven hours is also a requisite part of increasing your metabolism. If your sleeping pattern isn't good, your body won't function properly. When your body is tired, it will not have enough energy to burn off calories. When you do not sleep, you get stressed easily. When this happens, your body would release a wave of stress hormones which increases your appetite and also produces more fat. If you regularly exercise and have a normal diet, getting a good night's rest shouldn't be difficult.

Win the war against the bulge by incorporating all these simple alterations to your daily routine. Boosting your metabolism should never be a burden. Instead, view it as motivation so you would add a little more to your daily experiences but get the most out of life.

Getting your dream well-sculpted and super sexy body is something you may have aimed for many years. The first step to so losing enough weight is boosting your metabolic rate. After you've lost enough weight, you should draw up to a new goal; building a six pack. So many people will envy you as soon as you take off your shirt, but that's a story for another day.

CONCLUSION

So many public figures have been able to speed up their metabolic rate by making lifestyle changes. On her journey to weight loss, Khloe Kardashian adopted several techniques to increase her metabolic rate and burn fat and calories.

She had a complete transformation of diet and cut out carbs almost entirely from her diet. She powered up with proteins, and her daily diet consisted of eggs and oatmeal for breakfast, salads for lunch, fish or chicken and vegetables for dinner and fresh fruits in between. Protein has a high thermic effect, which means the body uses up more energy in digesting it which speeds up your metabolism.

She also opted for smaller servings multiple times throughout the day rather than one or two heavy meals. Like we established earlier, eating smaller portions increases your metabolic rate without overworking your body system.

Khloe infused a lot of fluid mainly water into her diet. When your body is dehydrated, it will lose energy, slow down metabolism and cause hunger and weakness. Water is the best fluid you can consume to get the metabolism boost without the extra calories and sugar you will find in soft drinks and juices. Khloe's final technique was regular exercise and an active lifestyle. Her trainer has admitted her dedication to going to the gym and remaining active even when she is not working out. Khloe engages in weight lifting, boxing, twisting lunges, squatting, jump ropes and taking walks. Her regular exercise routine is perhaps her most effective method to speed up her body's metabolism and build muscles. Khloe has been able to lose over 35 pounds in the past couple of months.

Actor Chris Pratt is another great example of weight and health transformation by increasing body metabolism. Pratt once weighed over 280 pounds and admitted to feeling less energetic and rundown. With a desire for transformation Pratt adopted a version of the Paleo diet in his meal plan. Similar to Khloe he almost completely cut out carbs and anything fried and consumed only proteins, fiber and lots of water for months. He ate more of fruits, vegetables, seeds, and nuts for fiber and ate lean meat and fish for protein. He also cut out all intake of alcoholic beverages, which can slow down body fat metabolism by as much as 73% for several hours. Chris began exercising regularly and did a highly intense triathlon training that included long periods of swimming, running and biking for months. In addition to this, he did weight lifting, crossfire high-intensity interval training, jogging, pull ups, pushups and just about any other activity that burnt energy and boosted his metabolism. Pratt was able to lose over 80 pounds in a couple of months and learned impulse control and discipline. He finished the 2015 Ironman 70.3 Florida triathlon impressively in 7 hours, 4 minutes and 52 seconds, and now feels more energetic and healthy every day.

When you start building a healthy lifestyle and reprogramming your taste buds. Over time, your brain will adjust to these healthier options. However, never underestimate the role exercise plays in boosting your metabolism. All these techniques are to help you kick start your metabolism indeed. Workout from time to time but do not work out too intensely and at the same time do not work out for too long at a time. Go easy, then gradually increase your speed. Small success would motivate you to keep going and reach the ultimate goal.

In no time, you would be able to jump start your metabolic rate. You'll feel much lighter, and you'll burn fat faster. Remember that understanding your metabolism should not be just about looking beautiful externally. It should be about being healthy internally and mentally as well. Make these changes part of your life. Don't just work on your metabolic rate because you want to lose weight for a party or a wedding. Do it because it is the right thing to do.

www.ingramcontent.com/pod-product-compliance
Lightning Source LLC
Chambersburg PA
CBHW070131290526
45789CB00005B/2201